A Beginner's Guide to Nutrition for Losing Weight

Easy-to-follow Nutrition Advice for weight Loss

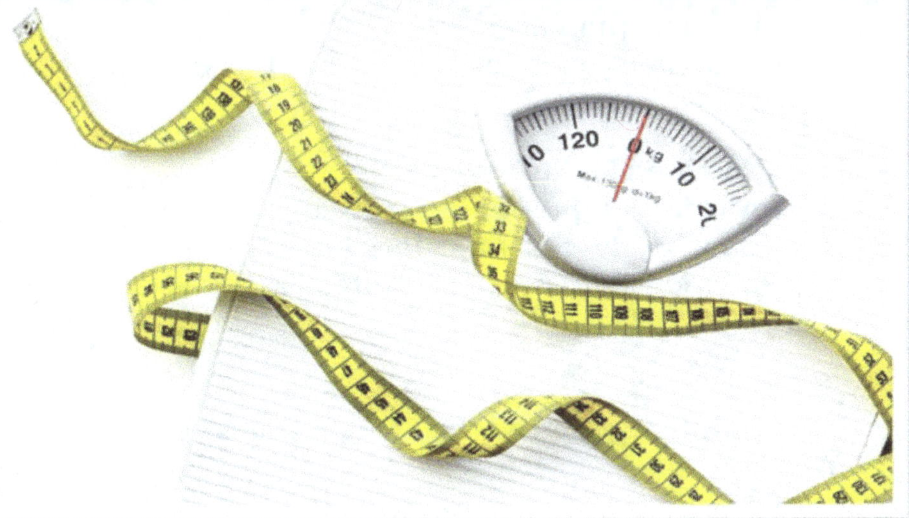

TABLE OF CONTENTS

$\mathbf{I}$ntroduction,

Burning fat, losing weight, getting in shape and looking great is easy ... when you eat healthy foods that make you feel fuller longer. Some foods naturally deliver a smaller calorie investment while giving your stomach a full feeling. You feel full, so you eat less, your calorie count goes down, and so does the size of your waistline. When you eat foods that provide little nutritional value with their calories, your mind tells you to eat more. It says, "Hey, we need nutrients, minerals and vitamins!" So you reach for more of the unhealthy food that is sitting in front of you. You eventually become full, but take in way more calories, fat and processed nasty than your body needs. The result? You pack on the weight and fat, your heart, circulatory system and entire body suffers, and you find yourself hungry again relatively quickly. Eat the following 10 healthy, nutritious types of foods that make you feel fuller longer, and you'll begin to lose weight as your whole body becomes healthier, and you begin to feel and look great.

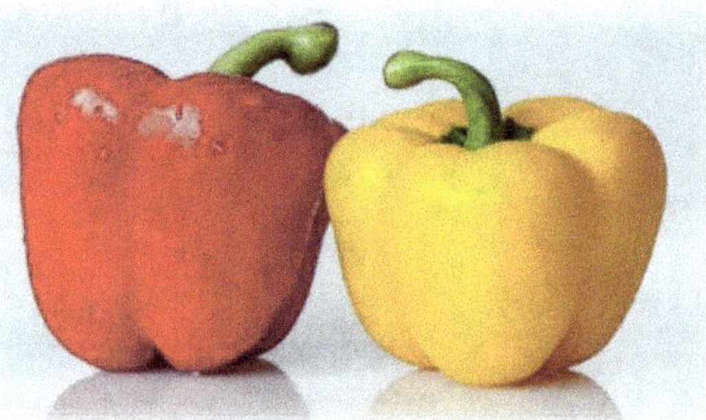

1 - Beans and Legumes.

"Beans, beans, the magical fruit; the more you eat, the more you toot!" That children's rhyme refers to the flatulence causing property of most beans. Yes, they can give you gas, no doubt about it. But on the marvelously positive side, they are extremely high in protein and dietary fiber. They can also fit into just about any budget and meal plan, since they are inexpensive and versatile. The FASEB Journal discovered in 2008 that if you eat just 4 ounces (1/2 cup) of beans a day, you bolster weight loss and weight maintenance. Beans are also a heart healthy food.

2 - Fresh Fruits.

Fresh fruits have a much lower energy density than milk, cheese, sweet foods and meats. This means they deliver fewer calories per gram, much fewer on a comparative basis. So you can eat several servings of super food fruits like blueberries, apples, bananas, blackberries, cantaloupes, citrus fruits, grapes, pomegranates and plums without paying much of a calorie penalty. And when you replace unhealthy, fat-filled, calorie-dense foods like potato chips, chocolate-bars and candy snacks with healthy fresh fruits, you double your fat-burning, weight loss effort.

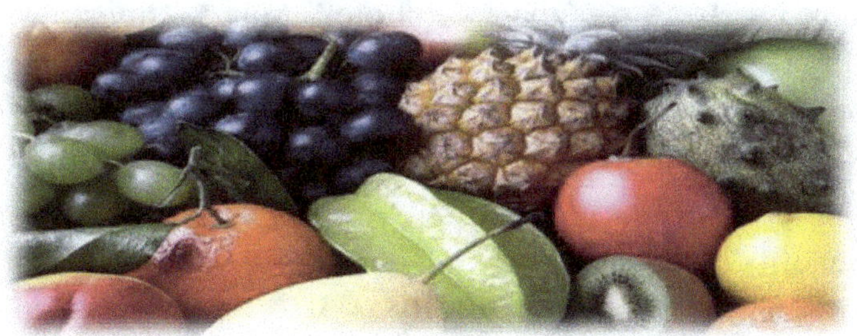

3 – Soups

Make sure you avoid store-bought soups, unless you are going to do some intelligent nutritional label research. A single can of soup that you purchase at your favorite grocery store often delivers several times your daily-recommended sodium allowance. Homemade soups give you total control over their contents. It is relatively easy to make a large batch of soup, and then portion off individual serving sizes that you can keep in your refrigerator and freezer for easy access. Soup is also easy on the budget, and because of its liquid base, quickly makes you feel full while delivering a limited number of calories.

4 - Fermented Foods

Do you like crunching down on a crisp, tart pickle? That's great, because fermented foods send a signal to your brain that starts a production of hormones that makes you feel full. This is true because of the short chain fatty acids (SCFAs) in foods that have been fermented, like kimchee, sauerkraut and pickles. A side benefit is the healthy probiotics found in most fermented foods. Probiotics are healthy bacteria that promote proper digestion. They actually live in your gut! Some health experts and physicians also believe that probiotics reduce your appetite. So enjoy some sauerkraut or pickles, and you will not only find yourself eating less, but your digestive system receives benefits as well.

5 – Eggs

Multiple studies show that when you eat protein with your breakfast, you ingest fewer calories throughout the day. Eggs are one of the healthiest sources of protein, and they also offer significant levels of vitamin B12, vitamin D and iron. The old, outdated belief that eggs were high in cholesterol has actually been explained in a little more detail in recent years. The type of cholesterol in eggs does not contribute to heart risks like most health professionals used to believe. This means you no longer need to worry about your egg intake. Eating 1 or 2 hard-boiled eggs between breakfast and lunch keeps you from overeating at your midday meal. And as we mentioned above, eating eggs for breakfast means you eat less during the day. A single large egg delivers 7 g of protein, 5 g of fat, just 1.6 g of saturated fat, and costs you only 75 calories. (See the recommended protein per pound of body weight formula at the end of this article to figure out exactly how much healthy, filling, low-calorie protein you need to eat every day.)

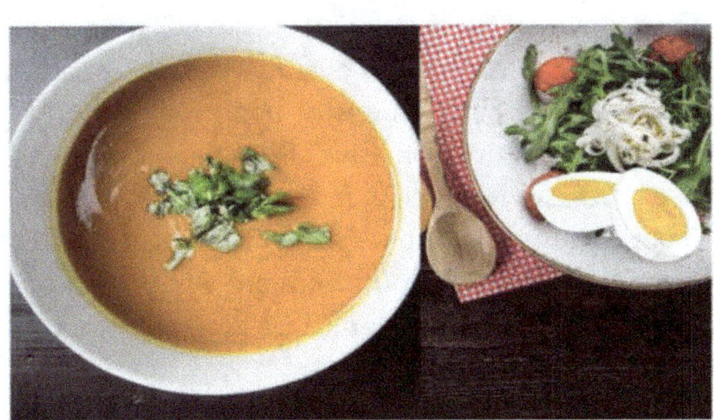

6 - Nuts and Nut Butters Nuts

Are packed full of healthy unsaturated fats. A healthy body needs fat, and the fats in nuts are just what you are looking for. On a per calorie basis, nuts and nut butters are extremely rich in fiber and protein. What are the 2 leading natural components that make you feel fuller longer? You guessed it, fiber and protein. Just don't eat too many nuts or too much nut butter at one sitting. Those healthy fats are in a very high quantity in nuts, and should not be over-consumed. So reach for a handful of almonds or walnuts the next time you are stuck between meals and craving something to eat. The heart healthy nature of nuts is just a wonderful side benefit of this versatile and tasty raw food.

7 - Broccoli and Brussels Sprouts

Repeat after me, "cruciferous vegetables". Vegetables like Brussels sprouts, broccoli and cauliflower belong to the cruciferous family. Cabbage, bok Choy, kale, collard greens and horseradish are also a part of this healthy vegetable subdivision. They deliver extremely high levels of healthy dietary fiber. As with other filling foods on this list, they are relatively inexpensive and extremely versatile, with most of them capable of being consumed raw or cooked. The antioxidants and cancer fighting ingredients in cruciferous foods are also worthy of note, and just another reason you need to be getting more of these healthy whole foods into your diet.

8 - Water

Okay, so water is not a food. We have to mention it anyway, because it is usually free or inexpensive, readily available, and is definitely required by the human body for proper maintenance and health. Did you know that the symptoms of thirst mimic those of hunger? That's right, so the next time you believe that you are hungry, drink 8 to 12 ounces of water. Give your body 10 minutes to process that liquid, and see how you feel then. You may truly be hungry. But the cranky mood, low energy and lack of ability to focus that often signals you are hungry may simply be telling you your body needs more liquids. Oh yeah, another big benefit of drinking water instead of eating anything? Zero calories.

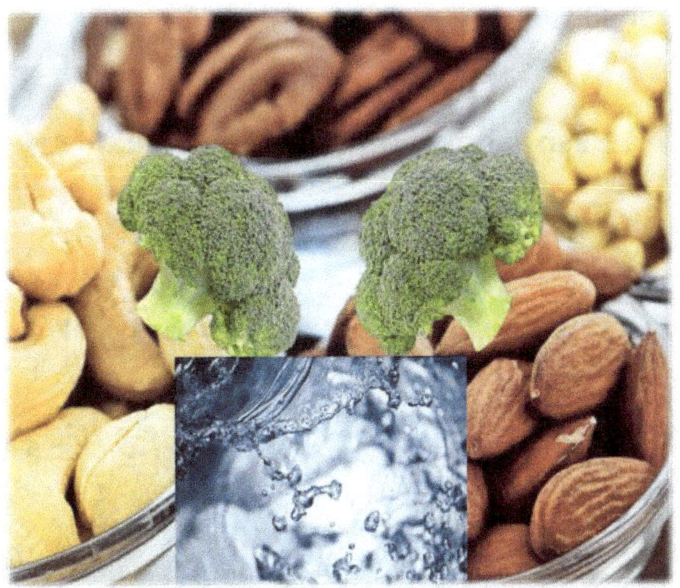

9 - Salmon, Anchovies and Tuna Fish

Helps you feel fuller longer while consuming fewer calories in a number of ways. First off, any type of fat will always help satisfy your hunger pangs. The types of fats found in high quantities in fish are essential fatty acids. Omega 3 EFAs are required by your body to function properly. Unfortunately, the human process does not create this healthy fat. You need to get it from outside sources, and fish like tuna and salmon have high levels of Omega 3s. That healthy fat makes you feel fuller longer, so you eat fewer calories during a fish-filled meal, as well as the rest of the day. Also, fish is packed full of wonderful protein. You have already seen earlier that protein satisfies hunger better than carbohydrates and fats. As if that is not good enough news, ocean caught salmon, anchovies and tuna are heart healthy foods as well.

10 - Raspberries, Blueberries, Blackberries

And Other Berries Most berries are extremely high in wonderful antioxidants that fight dangerous free radicals in your body. They are also extremely heart healthy, and deliver high levels of phytonutrients, minerals and vitamins that promote overall body health, inside and out. Your immunity system receives a huge boost when you eat berries regularly. This means that your natural defense system is much better prepared to ward off infections, disease and sickness. It also means that you recover from injuries and sickness quickly. Berries contribute a very small amount of calories considering the amount of filling fiber they deliver. Just 1 cup of raspberries offers a full 8 g of fiber. (The average adult needs between 25 and 30 g of dietary fiber each and every day from food items, not supplements.) Protein is the most satisfying type of food. More than carbohydrates and fats, protein satisfies your hunger more effectively than any other type of food. And guess what? Researchers are not even quite sure why protein acts like a stop sign, signaling your mind to stop eating. But it does, so make sure that you are getting the recommended 0.36 grams of protein per pound of body weight (about 0.8 grams of protein per kilogram) every day. And don't forget filling, healthy, digestive track regulating fiber. The "modern-day" diet is desperately lacking in dietary fiber. Foods like the brans, grains and oats listed above do a great job of delivering protein and dietary fiber, while limiting the amount of carbohydrates and calories you consume. To summarize, for a solution to burning fat, losing weight and maintaining a healthy body weight, eat foods high in fiber and/or protein. They have extremely high satiety index scores, which is a fancy way of saying they are healthy foods that make you feel fuller longer.

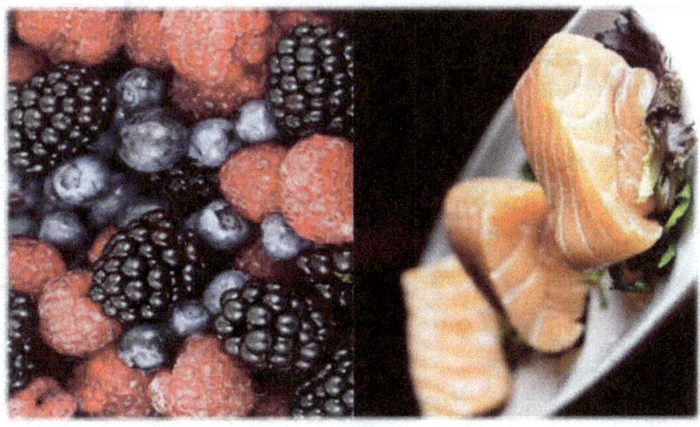

What is Good Nutrition?

Trying to eat better? It can be a confusing path. Information about what's healthy and how to lose weight comes in many shapes and forms, and the information is often contradictory. You might hear the old adage, "calories in, calories out." And the next minute you might read that "not all calories are equal."

So what's the truth and what is good nutrition? Do you trust the federal nutrition guidelines, your doctor, your best friend, the latest trend or do you listen to your body?

If you're confused and frustrated, you're not alone. The good news is that all of this confusion really only stems from two places:

1. New science and information being released
2. People trying to profit

These can overlap – quality companies and manufacturers do make good, nutritious food based on the latest in health and nutrition science. If you can evaluate the nutrition information you're reading or hearing and ask where the information comes from, then you're way ahead of the majority of the population. This guide incorporates that new science and information. We'll share what the guidelines are and why they have been created.

Let's start with the information you may have learned in grade school and how it's changed over the years.

The Basic Food Groups

Do you remember the food pyramid? Presently it looks a bit like this:

- 6-11 servings of bread, cereal, rice and pasta
- 3-5 servings of vegetables
- 2-3 servings of milk, yogurt, and cheese
- 2-3 servings of meat, eggs, nuts, eggs, beans
- Fats, oils, and sweets – use sparingly

It doesn't look like a big deal, right? You might look back on your day and think, "Well, I've had my six servings of grains and bread. I've had my dairy, meats and I've even had a fruit or veggie serving today. I'm not doing too badly."

Serving size matters! Servings are often misleading. For example, one serving of pasta is a half-cup of cooked pasta. Put that on your plate and you might frown because it looks like a quarter of what you might consider to be a serving. However, a serving of vegetables is a full cup. Serving size is where most people get tripped up. Why the difference? Why is a serving of pasta a half cup and a serving of vegetables a full cup? Because, while calories are equal mathematically, your body processes foods differently. Calories from a cookie are not the same as calories from an apple. Don't worry, we'll break it down so it's much easier for you to manage – you can eat nutritiously and lose weight.

Good Nutrition Helps You Lose Weight Because...

With all the fad diets and pills on the market you might wonder why nutrition matters. Many of the not so healthy foods we eat are inflammatory – that is, they make your tissues and cells swell up. This inflammation is responsible for most diseases, including heart disease, diabetes, and cancer.

It also causes weight gain.

Good nutrition reduces inflammation. Instead of constantly trying to repair, your body can function optimally. Good nutrition:

- Gives you more energy
- Increases your metabolism
- Repairs disease and dysfunction
- And much more.

Your body is an amazing machine. In many cases you can actually reverse damage done to it by simply changing your diet and fueling your body with the nutrition it needs and deserves. Before we dive into the nitty gritty, let's have a little fun and debunk some common nutrition myths.

Nutrition Myths – Busted!

Nutrition Myth #1 Carbs are bad

Carbohydrates are not inherently bad for you. In fact, they're one of the fastest sources of fuel for your body. However, all carbs are not created equally. A slice of white bread is much different than a slice of whole wheat bread. And white rice is different than brown rice. Whole grains generally have more fiber and more healthy fats.

Additionally, moderation is key here. Remember that a serving of pasta is ½ cup. If you have toast for breakfast, a sandwich for lunch, and a plate of pasta for dinner then you're probably consuming 7-9 servings of carbs and that's not including any chips or snacks you had during the day. These calories add up.

Here's the takeaway – eat carbs in moderation and pay attention to the type of carb you're eating.

Nutrition Myth #2 All Calories are Equal

You intuitively know this. You know that the calories you consume when you eat a pint of ice cream are not the same calories as you'd get from the caloric equivalent of vegetables. If you ate 1000 calories of veggies your body would burn them quickly and you'd take in a lot of nutrients. If you eat 1000 calories of ice cream your body stores those calories as fat.

Several studies have been conducted recently on this concept of "all calories are not created equally." One of the most notable studies placed 1600 people into three different diets. They found that the low fat diet had the worst results. The high protein high carb diet had great results in terms of weight loss but some unpleasant side effects, and it wasn't a diet people could stick to long term. However, the low glycemic diet – which favors whole foods rather than processed foods – had the best long-term results.

"It's time to reacquaint ourselves with minimally processed carbs. If you take three servings of refined carbohydrates and substitute one of fruit, one of beans and one of nuts, you could eliminate 50 percent of diet-related disease in the United States. These relatively modest changes can provide great benefit." David Ludwig, director of the study. You can find the details of this study at: http://opinionator.blogs.nytimes.com/2012/06/26/which-diet-works/?ref=opinion, or in the Journal of the American Medical Association at: http://jama.jamanetwork.com/article.aspx?articleid=119915 4.

Nutrition Myth #3 All Saturated Fat is Bad for You

For many years we were taught to believe that all saturated fat was bad for you. It raised cholesterol, caused heart disease and clogged our arteries. The truth is that there are different types of saturated fats and some of them are quite good for you.

"Researchers have long known that there are many kinds of saturated fats, and they are handled differently by the body when consumed. Stearic acid, a type of saturated fat found naturally in cocoa, dairy products, meats, and poultry, as well as palm and coconut oils, does not raise harmful LDL cholesterol but boosts beneficial HDL cholesterol levels." Source: Julie Upton, MS, RD, Cooking Light Magazine.

What is the takeaway from these three busted myths?

Good nutrition matters! Whole foods, foods found in nature, are the foundation of good nutrition. So now let's dive into the basic food groups and dig deep to discover why this is true and how good nutrition can help you change weight. Then we'll take a look at how to make changes in your daily habits to make good nutrition simple, easy, and a part of your life.

How Does Good Nutrition Help You Lose Weight?

What is good nutrition? We know it intuitively. We know that a box of macaroni and cheese isn't as nutritious as steamed broccoli. We know that a glass of water is better for us than a sugary coffee drink. But the choices aren't always that obvious are they? For example, what's better; a donut or a muffin?

Neither is ideal, however many would say that the donut is better because it has less sugar, fat, and even calories than the muffin.

For the sake of continuity and clarity let's define nutrition as the process of providing or obtaining the food necessary for health and growth.

And in this particular case, for weight loss. On that note, let's now explore the various aspects of good nutrition as they specifically help you lose weight.

Fiber

You hear it from doctors, nutritionists, and maybe even your mom. You need fiber in your diet. There are actually two types of fiber, and both are important – but in different ways.

Soluble fiber – this type of fiber can be broken down in water. It actually attracts water and forms a gel-like material in your stomach. Imagine eating a teaspoon of soluble fiber. It attracts and absorbs water and that teaspoon grows to about a quarter cup.

As you might imagine, that teaspoon of fiber creates a reaction that fills you up. Soluble fiber makes you feel full. This is how it helps you lose weight. You feel fuller, eat less, and consume fewer calories.

But what about insoluble fiber? It's fiber that is not broken down in your body. Insoluble fiber does not dissolve in water, which means it passes through your gastrointestinal tract relatively intact. This has the effect of bulldozing the passage of food and waste through your gut. You see, if food is allowed to sit in your gut it begins to attract bacteria. They feed on this stagnant material and guess what...you start to feel bloated. You'll also likely begin to feel lethargic as the bacteria multiply and begin to cause problems.

Insoluble fiber helps you lose weight because it keeps your digestive system running smoothly. It helps keep the balance of good bacteria in your stomach at optimal levels, and it reduces bloat and often increases your energy and sense of well-being.

So where do you find soluble and insoluble fiber?

As you might suspect, they come in the form of grains, fruits and vegetables. Here are a few food sources for both:

Sources of soluble fiber include:

- Oatmeal
- Lentils
- Apples
- Oranges
- Pears
- Strawberries
- Nuts
- Flaxseeds
- Beans
- Blueberries
- Cucumbers
- Celery
- Carrots

Sources of insoluble fiber include:

- Whole wheat
- Whole grains
- Wheat bran
- Seeds
- Nuts
- Barley
- Couscous
- Brown rice

- Bulgur
- Zucchini
- Celery
- Broccoli
- Cauliflower
- Cabbage
- Onions
- Tomatoes
- Carrots
- Green beans
- Dark leafy vegetables like spinach, kale, and collard greens

Start eating whole grains, more fruits and veggies and not only will the weight begin to come off, you'll feel better too.

Inflammation

Your body responds to toxins, poisons, viruses, injury, and invaders through inflammation. It's a process that actually strives to bring more nourishment and immune activity to a site of injury or infection – wherever that infection may be. If you sprain your ankle, your ankle will swell in a protective response. When your cells are irritated the same thing happens.

Biologically this is usually a good response. Unfortunately, there are many things in our modern diet that cause chronic inflammation. They're perceived by our bodies as toxins and poisons. The result is a state of chronic inflammation, which has been shown to lead to the majority of deadly diseases we're dealing with today. These diseases include heart disease, diabetes, Alzheimer's, cancer and much more. It also causes obesity.

Reduce, or eliminate, these inflammatory foods and you'll not only reduce your risk of these serious diseases, you'll lose weight. So what are the foods you should eat?

Let's first take a look at the primary foods that cause inflammation:

- Sugar – Any type of sugar causes inflammation. Cane sugar isn't better than high fructose corn syrup here. Sugar causes inflammation.
- White flour – Your body treats white flour and starchy carbohydrates much like sugar. It's processed quickly, causes a spike in blood sugar and leads to inflammation.
- Trans fats – Trans fats are the bad fats found in cakes, pastries, margarine, and shortening, among other foods. Avoid them completely.

So what can you eat that will reduce inflammation?

You already know this – look at your food pyramid. Fruits, vegetables, whole grains, and healthy fats are all okay. Other things like green tea, fish rich in Omega-3 fatty acids and nuts all help reduce inflammation and help you lose weight.

Metabolism

Your metabolism is the process that provides energy to your cells. It powers every thought, action, and movement you make. Your body needs energy to survive and thrive. When you provide it with nutritious foods that fuel your body, it can run smoothly like a car with the optimal grade of fuel in it. However, when you fuel your body in an unhealthy manner, your body has to fight and struggle to extract nutrients from that food and to battle any negative response. You may generate a little energy from junk food, but it comes at a great cost. However, with nutritious foods you generate energy only – no extra cost to your body. Thus, you can eat less and feel better. You'll lose weight.

Some foods are known for boosting your metabolism. They include:

- Lean protein – fish is particularly good for your metabolism and it has healthy Omega-3 fatty acids to reduce inflammation.
- Green tea – full of anti-oxidants and a small bit of caffeine. It has been shown to increase metabolism and reduce risks of certain cancers.

Broccoli, grapefruit, and high fiber foods including fruits, vegetables, and whole grains. You may see a trend here – fruits, vegetables, and whole grains are some easy foods to focus on. Replace some of your unhealthy foods with vegetables and fruits and you're on the right path.

Steady Blood Sugar Levels

The food you eat has an impact on your blood sugar. For example, place a bit of sugar in your mouth and you might notice that it begins dissolving and digesting almost immediately. Foods that have a high glycemic level are digested quickly and cause a spike in your blood sugar levels. This isn't a big problem if it only happens occasionally.

However, the modern diet causes your blood sugar to spike multiple times every day. Each time you eat a sugary, starchy snack you're causing your blood sugar to spike. Unfortunately, what goes up must come down, including your blood sugar. This leaves you feeling exhausted and craving foods that will give you another quick blood sugar spike. All of this up and down is hard on your body.

You're not only eating more food than your body needs, and thus storing fat, you're also causing your insulin system to become resistant. This means that it stops hearing the signals from your body and it takes more and higher glycemic foods to give you the energy you need.

Foods that are high in sugar and starchy carbohydrates are the biggest offenders, meaning they cause the highest blood sugar spikes.

Avoid:

- French fries
- Sugary drinks
- Bagels
- Pretzels
- White rice
- White potatoes
- Cereal

So what can you have? You might already know the answer to this question based on the trends in the previous guidelines. Yep, you guessed it; fruits, vegetables, and whole grains.

Low glycemic foods stabilize blood sugar and include:

- Artichokes
- Eggplant
- Asparagus
- Green beans
- Peppers
- Squash
- Spinach
- Kale
- Collards
- Tomatoes
- Carrots
- Sweet potatoes
- Zucchini
- Apples
- Pears

- Peaches
- Kiwi
- Oranges
- Nuts and seeds
- Beans and lentils
- Oats
- Quinoa
- Millet

Many experts also recommend dairy and/or soy products as low glycemic options. Take care if you have allergies or sensitivities to dairy or soy – many people find that they have issues with these foods, which can then cause inflammation.

So now you have a solid understanding of how nutrition can impact your health and your weight. However, at this point you may still feel overwhelmed. The remainder of this report is dedicated to helping you not only create a plan to overhaul your diet and change your live but to guide you on how to make those changes as easy and painless as possible.

Make Small Changes – Reap Big Results

Deciding to eat healthier is the first step to losing weight and keeping it off for the rest of your life. If you've made that decision then you're halfway there. The second step is to commit to changing your habits, one at a time.

Sure, it's tempting to want to make a huge change. Unfortunately, few can make that kind of life overhaul stick for the long term. Instead, it's much easier to tackle one habit at a time. It's also more powerful. You can systematically identify the nutritional and food challenges you personally face and create a lifestyle that fits your needs. Many "diets" are created with a "one size fits all" approach. The problem is that you have a unique body with its own systems and sensitivities.

For example, gluten may cause you to have some stomach issues, but you may not know that until you begin to change how you eat. You may realize that the carbs you can eat need to be very different from the carbs that the FDA recommends.

Let's take a look at the process of changing your life, one habit at a time, and adopting a healthier and more nutritious lifestyle for lasting weight loss.

The Power of Changing Your Habits

First, take a deep breath and relax. Good nutrition isn't a "diet." It's not about going on some highly regimented plan for a few months and hoping for the best. Rather, you're changing your lifestyle for lasting health and sustained weight loss. Here's how:

Step One: Identify Poor Nutrition Habits

There's no room for shame here. Sit down, be honest with yourself and start listing the dietary and nutrition habits you need to change. Let's step back to that food pyramid for a second.

- How many fruits and vegetables do you eat each day?
- Do you eat breakfast and if so, what do you eat?
- Do you drink your calories (e.g., soda, juice and sugary coffee drinks or sports drinks)?
- What do you snack on?
- Do you eat whole grains?
- Do you eat processed foods?
- How much fat and sugar do you eat daily?

Start making a list of the habits you want to change. Prioritize the list. What's the first habit to change? It might be the one that's the easiest to change or it might be the one that you feel will have the biggest impact.

For example, you might decide to switch to whole grain bread instead of white bread. That's a simple step that's pretty easy to take. Or you might decide to start having a morning breakfast smoothie. This smoothie could contain half your day's fruits and veggies. It would significantly impact your health and nutrition in a positive way but might require you to make some changes to your morning routine – in short, it might not be easy, but it will be worth it.

So decide the habit you want to tackle first and decide how you're going to replace that unhealthy habit with a nutritious one. Make a plan.

Tackle Your Habits One at a Time

They say it takes about 21 days to create a new habit. So that gives you about three weeks for each new habit. Take this time. Give yourself room to adapt and grow. You can get overwhelmed by trying to make too many changes at once. You may begin feeling restricted and deprived. Then what usually happens is a backlash. You might be doing well for several weeks as you cut out all of those unhealthy habits and hold yourself to a very high standard. But then you have a bad day, something stresses you out, you fall back into old habits and all of that hard work is forgotten.

When you give yourself time to adapt and change you won't feel deprived. You won't feel overwhelmed, and you won't lose control. And when you do have a soda, eat an ice cream sundae or enjoy a cheeseburger you won't feel like you've failed because you know that you're in control and one "cheat" does not ruin all of your efforts for the day, nor will it impact how you eat tomorrow.

Eating healthy isn't about being perfect. It's about knowing what foods fuel your body and make you feel great. You'll lose weight, it'll stay off, and you'll be able to enjoy the occasional indulgence without feeling guilty or like you failed.

And here's a side benefit that might surprise you...

With each change you make, you'll gather momentum. So next, let's take a look at some small changes you can make to get big results.

Small Changes You Can Make To Get Big Results

- Kick the soda habit.
- Eat fruits and veggies for snacks.
- Eat a healthy breakfast!
- No more starchy carbs. Start replacing them with whole grains.
- Veggies with every meal – including breakfast.
- Bring your own lunch to work – it's difficult to eat a nutritious meal at most restaurants.

- Eat fish at least once a week.
- Eat a vegetarian dinner once a week.
- Try a new fruit or vegetable weekly.
- Bring snacks with you – don't allow yourself to get to the point where you're so hungry you're craving sugar or junk.
- Drink more water and fewer sugary drinks like juice or coffee drinks.

Remember, it's much easier and you have a better chance of success when you tackle one habit at a time. Start with the habit that makes the most sense for you, create a plan to make it happen and enjoy the results. Before we wrap up, here's a quick example of how you might create a plan for one of these habits.

Let's say you have a habit of drinking soda during the day. You know they're empty calories with no nutritional value whatsoever and diet soda isn't much better. So you decide that's the habit you want to replace first. You'll need a two-pronged approach. How will you quit drinking soda and what good habit will you replace it with?

If you drink several sodas a day you might cut back to one per day for a few days and then half a soda a day for a few days and then just one soda a week. You could replace your soda with water or even carbonated water. After a week or two of drinking one soda a week, it'll be easy to quit drinking soda all together. If you drink two sodas a day, simply quitting this habit will help you lose a pound a week or 52 pounds in a year! Small changes reap huge rewards!

Getting Started

As you begin to make changes to your nutritional habits and start losing weight remember that this is supposed to be a positive and fun experience. Stay focused on your long-term goal, which is to get healthy and to look and feel better.

Don't feel like the food you have to eat needs to be tasteless to be nutritious – real food is delicious, and weight loss and good nutrition can be too. Stay focused on your long term goals and when you make mistakes, don't give up. Keep working to modify your nutritional habits to live a long and healthy life at your ideal weight.

A Beginner's Guide to Balancing the Food Groups

When trying to lose weight, it's hard at first to know what to eat. You want to make sure you're not hungry – a downfall to any diet – but you also don't want to jeopardize your weight loss by eating too much. So how do you find a happy medium? You do it by balancing your food groups.

Let's Get Visual

Let's break this concept of balancing food groups down into a visual. Take a look at your plate and divide it in half. Fill one half of it with vegetables and fruit. Now, split the other half in two and fill one side with a meat or a high quality protein choice like eggs, cottage cheese, or legumes. The remaining portion of your plate can be completed with a whole grain choice like a hearty multi grain bread or other complex carbohydrate.

Breakfast

In taking a look at your day, let's take define what each meal and snack should look like. For breakfast, you always want to have a high protein meal because it sets your body into fat burning mode right away and also keeps hunger pangs at bay longer. Greek yogurt is very high in protein and has thick consistency to it, making it an ideal and filling choice to start your day. If you are lactose intolerant, have a couple of eggs. Add a cup of fresh fruit and a slice of whole grain toast and a handful of almonds or walnuts and you are off to a good start to your day.

Morning Snack

A handful of vegetables like carrots or a small bunch of grapes with a slice of low fat cheese or perhaps a couple of tablespoons of peanut butter or hummus will keep you full and humming along into your lunch hour.

Lunch

Make the majority of this meal vegetables. Vegetable soup, salad, or just a mixture of fresh vegetables and low fat dip should be the foundation of what you eat. Add three ounces of lean meat like chicken without the skin, lean beef, or legumes if you are vegetarian, plus a few whole grain crackers, and you have enough healthy protein and fiber to fill you until late afternoon.

Dinner

Again, this meal should be half a plate of vegetables – say, tossed green salad with a sweet potato on the side – and then a cut of lean meat or fish and you have another successful meal sitting in front of you.

A Guide to Carbohydrates and Weight Loss
Carbohydrates are nutrients

That your body breaks down to create sugar. Like other nutrients, carbohydrates also provide vitamins and minerals. But what does this have to do with losing weight?

Why Does the Body Need Sugar?

The cells in our body use sugar to make energy and your brain runs off of it exclusively for fuel. So, just like gas for your car, carbohydrates keeping the motor running. And while it is also true your body can run off fat and protein for a while, it will eventually need to switch back to carbohydrates, otherwise it will start eating its own muscle for fuel – not a good idea when dieting since it lowers your overall rate at which your body burns calories.

Two Kinds of Fuel

There are two types of carbohydrates: simple and complex. Simple carbohydrates are easily absorbed and provide quick energy to the body. Have you ever reached for a candy bar when you were feeling tired? That's you feeding your body simple carbohydrates to get the boost you needed. More examples of simple carbohydrates are honey, breakfast cereals, breads and biscuits made with white flour, fruit juice, and most crackers. Complex carbohydrates aren't as quickly digested as your body since they usually contain fiber and as a result, don't cause the spikes in blood sugar. They also carry a lot more nutrients than simple sugars. Some examples of complex carbohydrates include whole grains, fruits, vegetables, and legumes. There has been a lot of talk about carbohydrates and how they hinder weight loss. To a certain extent that is true – if you eat too many carbs, then your body will end up storing them as fat. In addition, when you continue to go overboard on carbs, you become sluggish, overweight and retain water. But here's the thing: your body needs carbohydrates to fuel your brain, to create red blood cells (a key component of blood) and to repair wounds. So how much is too much? Recent scientific studies show that daily carbohydrate intake between 100 grams and 150 grams per day is right where you want to be; enough carbs to run your body in a healthy, efficient manner but not get in the way of weight loss. Of course, if you are exercising strenuously on a daily basis, are recovering from illness or surgery, or have other health issues like diabetes, your optimum carbohydrate intake level may be different – and in some case, dramatically different. It's best to check with your doctor to be sure.

A Guide to the 6 Nutrients Your Body Needs On A Daily Basis

For your body to function properly, you need to give your body six essential nutrients each day. Here's a quick overview of each one.

Water

Water is the most basic nutrient your body needs. Every single cell in your body needs it to function and up to 70% of our body is made up of water. It helps regulate our body temperature and heartbeat, helps the cells deliver energy and is vital in burning fat, just to name a few functions. Most experts recommend 7-8 glasses of water a day in addition to the five servings of fruits and vegetables we should be eating. Anything with caffeine in it does not count toward your recommended daily allotment since caffeine drinks like coffee and tea expel water from the body?

Minerals

Minerals like magnesium are involved in over 500 distinct processes in the body; sodium and potassium help keep your heart beat regular and calcium is essential for not only your bones but for your muscles, too. Eating a wide variety of vegetables, especially dark leafy greens, will help provide the daily intake you need.

Vitamins

Vitamins are chemical components that help other chemical reactions happen in our bodies. Involved in almost every function in our body, from our immune system to our mood levels to our bone strength, vitamins make our bodies' functions possible. Since cooking destroys certain vitamins, it is best to eat the majority of your food raw, steamed, grilled, or stir-fried to get the most benefit from the available vitamins in your food.

Protein

Without protein, our bodies couldn't manufacture the amino acids needed to repair muscle tissue, or control certain hormones properly. It is also used as a source of energy when there are not enough carbohydrates available. Good sources of protein include eggs, fish, chicken, beef, milk, beans and seeds.

Carbohydrates

The fuel that is the body's first choice in running the brain and the muscles, carbohydrates play an important role in the everyday functioning of what makes us who we are. There are two classes of carbohydrates: simple and complex. Simple carbohydrates like honey, refined grains, and candy provide almost instant energy boost that doesn't last long. Complex carbohydrates, on the other hand, provide the body fuel as well, but also depart a more sustained source of energy, avoiding those highs and lows. Foods that should be considered as good carbohydrate sources are vegetables, legumes, nuts and seeds.

Fats

While scorned upon in the diet world, fats are absolutely essential to the functioning of our bodies. Our nerve fibers are sheathed in particular type of fat which enables the electric signals to travel properly. Our brains are mostly fat, helping us to think quickly. And our organs are cushioned by fat, protecting them from sudden jarring and in other cases, providing an emergency source of fuel when the rest of the fat storage has run out. Healthy sources of fat include olive oil, salmon, walnuts, and fish oil.

Do Antioxidants Help Weight Loss?

You hear the word antioxidant a lot when people talk about health. But what exactly are antioxidants and how can they help with weight loss? The way your body burns fuel is very similar to the way a fire in a fire place burns. There needs to be fuel and oxygen for the fire to start and to continue burning. Once the fire has died out, there is ash and soot left behind in the fireplace. In our bodies, fuel and oxygen are needed to produce the energy we need and once the process is done, there is residue left over, just like in the fire place. This residue is known by the name of oxidants. And just like soot in the fireplace, if oxidants aren't cleaned up, the result can be disastrous. A healthy body is capable of cleaning up the normal load of oxidants. It does this by using antioxidants which clean the reside from the body and prevent from becoming an irritant and damaging other nearby cells. However, when we eat a lot junk food, don't exercise, don't drink enough water and live with an elevated level of stress consistently, the body is unable to remove the oxidants as efficiently as it should. If the body is overwhelmed with the oxidant level on a daily basis, then cells and tissues within the body start to deteriorate, setting up the environment for shortened cell life, lowered immune system functions, and general rapid aging of the entire body. Being overweight generates a low but persistent level of inflammation in the body which adds to already unmanageable levels of oxidant activity. Your body is in a state of disrepair and cannot fix itself properly. That means losing weight is even harder because your body sees it as another form of stress. There is a way to combat oxidative stress - certain foods have the ability to stop the corrosive oxidative effect and thus are called antioxidants.

These foods - most of them fruits - excel at sweeping up the residue as well as stopping the chain of deterioration oxidants create. Making sure to include at least two cups of the following foods in your diet every day will go a long way in lowering the stress level of your body, allowing to heal and to release fat as it improves it fuel burning capabilities.

Those foods are:

* Blueberries * strawberries * prunes * blackberries * red delicious apples * Granny Smith apples * plums * raspberries * sweet cherries * black, red kidney, or pinto beans Eat and enjoy the weight loss!

Do You Need Weight Loss Supplements?

Losing weight involves a lot of change in your body – and not just in you're eating and exercise habits. Internally, changing how your body goes about burning energy as well as how much energy it burns can be a time-consuming process. In this day and age of instant results, it's no surprise there are weight loss supplements to speed up the process of shedding weight, whether you are just starting your diet or have hit a plateau in your weight loss journey. How do you know when you need a weight loss supplement? This can vary from person to person, but a general rule of thumb is when you have stalled at a particular weight for more than a month and have both increased your exercise as well as been true to your calorie goals, then you may want to think about a weight loss supplement. The most important thing in deciding to use a supplement is talk to your doctor first. Why? There may be other reasons why you are not losing weight and your doctor may pick up on a change in your health that needs addressed. Weight loss supplements can range from fiber supplements to meal replacements to herbs to man-made chemicals that increase the metabolism. Generally speaking, only a handful of supplements have any official track record of increasing weight loss. They most proven and reliable supplements are fiber and meal replacements.

Fiber

Dietary fiber, sometimes called roughage, is the part of food from plants that is indigestible by our gastric systems. Fiber – either through powder, capsule, or food -

slows the digestive process down and makes you feel fuller. Fiber also acts as a type of broom as it moves through your intestines, collecting leftover debris and sweeping it out of the body, aiding in weight loss that normally isn't addressed through exercise or calorie reduction. Be careful not to increase fiber too rapidly as it will cause bloating and gas as your intestines are cleaned out. Also be sure to drink two to three more glasses of water each day as you gradually increase your fiber intake so you do not become constipated.

Meal Replacements

Meal replacements – whether in the form of a bar, a shake, or a pre-made meal – really do work if you follow along with the plan. Usually, you substitute breakfast and lunch with the meal replacements and have a snack of fruit or other low calorie item and then around a 500 calorie dinner. When combined with consistency of maintaining caloric goals and exercising regularly, it really does help you lose weight.

Essential Vitamins and Minerals For Weight Loss

While we all need to intake vitamins and minerals every day to remain healthy, weight loss can be helped along by ensuring we have adequate intake of a few particular nutrients. This is especially important considering in the past 20 years, modern farming practices have consistently produced food that, while plentiful and attractive to the eye, have 80% less nutritional value than they did a generation or two ago.

Chromium

Chromium is mineral that stabilizes blood sugar levels, decreasing the likelihood of sudden waves of hunger, mood swings, and binging. In the long term, it works to prevent diabetes and heart disease because of its leveling effect. You can take chromium as a supplement but it is always best to obtain it through foods such as corn, sweet potatoes, apples, eggs, tomatoes, and broccoli.

Magnesium

Surprisingly little emphasis is placed by the media on the role the mineral magnesium plays in weight loss. Magnesium plays critical parts in food digestion, insulin regulation (insulin determines whether energy is used or stored as fat), and controlling the body's chemical reactions to stress, which causes weight gain. Food sources of magnesium include rice, wheat, and oat bran, pumpkin seeds, spinach, flax, sesame seeds, Brazil nuts, almonds, sunflower seeds, molasses and edamame (dry roasted soybeans).

Zinc

Here is another key player in the weight loss game: the mineral zinc helps control metabolism and lean muscle mass as well as the immune system, so this is one mineral to pay attention to. Quick tip: you can tell if you are zinc deficient by looking at your finger nails. If there are white spots, then that is a usually reliable indicator that you are lacking zinc in your diet. You can always take zinc in a supplemental form, but getting it from food sources is a much better route to take. Zinc can be found in oysters, toasted wheat germ, roasted pumpkin seeds, low fat roast beef, peanuts, crab, and lamb.

Vitamin D

Once just thought of as being useful for strong bones, Vitamin D is becoming a major force in the nutritional world, including the weight loss arena. Adequate amounts of this vitamin help transition the body metabolism from fat storing to fat burning and has the additional benefit of burning belly fat first. Vitamin D is made by exposing the skin to sunlight each day. While this is not always possible, you can take an oral supplement Vitamin D to ensure your body is maintaining proper levels.

Good Fats vs. Bad Fats

For Weight Loss let's start with the basic truth about fat: it is absolutely essential to our bodies. It cushions our organs, helps assimilate certain vitamins, provides fuel for energy and most importantly, is essential to our brains – they are 60% fat! Plus, eating a little fat at every meal slows the digesting process down and keeps us feeling fuller, longer.

Now that we've established that fat is a critical to the well-being your body, let's see how it fits into your diet. It's important to know that there are three types of fat in your food – saturated, unsaturated and Trans fat - and only one of those types will help you lose weight by keeping you feeling full and maintaining your health. The key to fat intake and weight loss is to make sure you don't eat more than 30% of your daily calorie allowance in fat.

The Two Kinds of Bad Fats

Saturated fat is usually found in red meat, full fat dairy products such as butter, milk and cheese as well as in palm and palm kernel oils. So what makes it bad? It has been linked to inflammation in our bodies, which means it creates a continuously unhealthy environment that can lead to heart disease, cancer, and other illnesses. Limiting consumption red meat to once a week and using low-fat or fat free dairy products helps to control your weight and the inflammation.

Tran's fats are man-made fats. Manufacturers found that this fat greatly extended the shelf life of baked goods like bread, cookies, and crackers and began incorporating it into the majority of foods we see today. The drawback? Our bodies can't handle it. Because it is a man-made chemical, the human body doesn't have the ability to break it down properly so it tries to store it, resulting in weight gain, inflammation and eventually, disease. Tran's fats are also known to contribute to clogging up arteries. Extra tip: Trans fats can also be listed as 'partially hydrogenated fat' on food labels, so if you see that phrase, don't eat it.

The Good Fat

So what fats are good for you and your waistline? Unsaturated fat. Your body recognizes this type of fat as easily absorbable and containing useful nutrients. Examples of this type of fat are found in foods like olive oil, almonds, avocados, peanuts, walnuts, seeds, spinach, kale, and flax oil. Cold water fish like salmon, tuna, mackerel, sardines, and herring also contain unsaturated fat. Eating these types of food will keep you feeling full and keep your body healthy.

How Small Efforts In Portion Control Can Achieve Weight Loss

When embarking on a weight loss diet, it's easy to think about all the big steps that need to be taken regarding portion control and food: counting calories, keeping track of fat grams, eating enough fiber, etc. It's easy to get overwhelmed. Yet, if you take it one small step at a time, you can break this portion control effort into easily handled steps.

Start Planning

The easiest way to get a handle on portion control is to set aside one day out of the week and plan your menu. Nothing too detailed, unless you need it to be that way - just quickly jot down what you think you will eat for each meal and snack. At that point, grab your plastic sandwich bags and your food storage containers and set aside how many you will need for each meal, each day: two sandwich bags for snacks, three storage containers for meals. Why? Because when you prepackage your food for school or work, you take away the danger of mindless overeating. You can do the same for food at home, too. You may have saved money buying the family-sized bag of pretzels but if you end up eating the whole thing in one sitting, you find the cost of it staring back at you from the scale numbers as you weigh yourself. So portion out your snacks at home, too. It will save you from unnecessary temptation.

Be Mindful of What You Eat

When you are eating out, a small but effective way to control portions is to ask for a doggie bag to be brought out with your meal. That way, you can quickly put half of the meal away for later and concentrate on eating what's in front of you, which is more likely to be a proper portion anyway.

Here's another super easy trick: know the serving size of your favorite treat. Then prepackage it. Is it a handful of chocolate candies? A half cup of that rich ice cream? Or maybe just a thin slice of cheesecake? Denying yourself is never a good idea when trying to lose weight. It seems contradictory, but when you give yourself a (little) treat while dieting, you will have a better chance of sticking to your weight loss program. The key is to know the size of a single serving, and then make sure it's ready on hand to have when the urge to indulge strikes. The best of dieting intentions can go awry when we are having one of those 'weak' moments.

How To Modify Recipes For Healthier Results

Craving the creamy, dreamy taste of mashed potatoes but can't indulge because you are on a diet? Or are you more of a sweet tooth type, thinking of the decadent sweetness of a brownie but can't indulge? Well, with a few quick and easy substitutions, you can still relish your favorite foods without totally falling off the diet wagon.

Substituting Fats

When it comes to making things taste good, fat does a really good job. Let's take a look at a some substitutes you can use when trying to reduce the impact of fat in your weight loss journey.

Plain Greek yogurt: many people don't yet realize the versatility of this particular dairy product. Thick, creamy and high in protein, nonfat or low fat plain Greek yogurt is an excellent substitute for sour cream on your baked potato or in your mashed potatoes. In casseroles, replacing cream of chicken soup with Greek yogurt really knocks down the calorie count without sacrificing the creamy texture or taste.

Applesauce: this humble food is a terrific substitute for fat when making baked goods like brownies. Most brownie and other bake mixes call for at least a 1/3 cup of oil in the recipe. That's over 330 calories just in the oil itself - not to mention the whopping 34 grams of fat. When replacing oil with applesauce, measure 1/4 cup of applesauce's for every 1/3 cup of oil. The best part of this substitution is that your baked goods - either cakes or brownies - won't have any flavor of the applesauce whatsoever.

Low fat and non-fat cheese: who doesn't love a little cheese? But that cheesy goodness comes with a price - high fat and calories. Thankfully, the dairy industry has risen to the call of the dieters and has come up with tasty, lower fat versions of its usual fat-filled fare. Substitutions are easy: use the low fat cheese exactly the same as you would normal cheese in your casseroles, eggs, and other foods. One word of caution: nonfat cheese doesn't melt nearly as well as low fat cheese and is best used for sprinkling in salads and on top of soups and stews.

Substituting Sweets

There are several substitutes on the market when it comes to replacing sugar with something a little lower calorie. The artificial sweetener saccharin is good for drinks and sprinkling on top of fruits, yogurts and hot cereals but it does not do well in baking. Each individual serving packet has less than four calories but contains the sweetness of two teaspoons of sugar. Sucralose, another artificial sweetener, has the same sweetness as saccharin but can be used in baking. Since it is not metabolized by the body, it has no calories. Aspartame has the same sweetness level as saccharin and sucralose and can be used in recipes, but they must be custom-made for aspartame use.

How To Understand The Nutritional Value of Every Day Foods and Packaged Foods

Every bite you eat impacts your health – with each swallow you are either moving toward your weight goal or away from it. So how do you figure out what to eat and how much to eat of it every day? You can calculate this information from reading the nutrition labels on foods.

Serving Size

On the label, the serving size is listed first. The rest of the information on the label is based on the serving size, so it's important to look closely at it. Is the whole package one serving? Or is it showing the data for one serving but the package is actually three servings? It's easy to glance at a bag of chips and think 'Oh, it's only 100 calories' when in reality it is really 300 calories for the entire bag.

Percent of Daily Value

The percent of daily value is calculated for a 2,000 calorie day. The nutrient guidelines tell you how much percentage of each nutrient is in the food when compared to that 2,000 calories. As you read through labels, keep these numbers in the back of your mind:

Total grams of fat intake per day should be somewhere between 56 – 78 grams (for a 2,000 calorie daily diet). So, if you eat a serving of food that has 10 grams of fat listed, you just ate 15% of your allotted amount of fat for the day.

Total amount of sodium per day should be no more than 2,400 milligrams. It seems like a lot until you start looking at labels, especially for foods like ketchup, soup, soda pop, and bread. It adds up quickly!

As you look at the vitamins and minerals listed on the labels, you naturally want to strive towards reaching at least 100% of your daily recommended allowance since that is minimum benchmark for maintaining health.

A 'Handy' Guide to Portion Size

Now that you know about reading food labels, how do you know when you have a good portion size? Look at your hand. Make a fist. That is about one cup of salad, fresh fruit, casserole, or drink. A cupped hand is about ½ cup serving size. That one is really good for measuring rice, pasta, potatoes, or ice cream. Your palm holds about three ounces, which is one single serving size of meat. Your thumb approximates one tablespoon – good for measuring salad dressings and sour cream. And finally, the tip of your thumb is equal to a teaspoon – perfect for butter, oil, and mayonnaise.

How You Eat Your Food Is Just As Important As What You Eat

A lot of focus is put on what you eat while you are dieting. But how you eat is just as important and can help you lose weight. What does that mean exactly?

Let's start with the biology of that statement. When you sit down to a meal and start to eat, it will be twenty minutes before your brain receives the signal that you have eaten enough to be full. So if you eat quickly and eat a lot, chances are twenty minutes after the start of your meal, you will be getting the feeling that you ate too much - you went beyond what your body needed to feel satiated.

A lot of times this happens when we eat in the car or standing in front of the TV. In other words, not sitting down in a relaxed manner, getting ready to enjoy a meal. So the first step in slowing down your eating to lose weight is to sit down and take a moment to relax. Even in the car, you can consciously slow your pace of eating to bring yourself more awareness of your meal. Once you've become aware of your pace, be mindful of it for the next twenty minutes and give your brain a chance to register the food.

Chewing slowly can also help you lose weight. How? Digestion actually begins in your mouth, not in your stomach. Certain enzymes in your saliva start breaking down simple carbohydrates while your teeth work to grind and tear apart more complex food molecules. The part of digestion is incredibly important to weight loss because the more thoroughly we chew our food, the more nutrients we extract, the more efficient our bodies run and the less cravings we have. Since it takes time to chew, you will most likely hit that 20 minute mark naturally and at the point of true fullness. Recent studies show that volunteers who chewed each mouthful forty times ended up eating twelve percent less food. That's enough to put a downward dent in the scale. And it all begins in your mouth!

Getting into the habit of eating slowing and chewing more thoroughly can be a little challenging at first. If you have trouble remembering to do so, try this little trick: put your fork down in between each bite. Consciously stopping the momentum of feeding yourself can be key to setting this practice into a consistent daily routine.

The 3 Top Reasons To Eat A Healthful Balanced Diet

While weight loss is the primary reason people choose to eat a healthy, balanced diet there are other benefits as well. A balanced diet incorporates the right amount of the right foods, eaten consistently for a properly functioning mind and body and when you eat this way on a daily basis, it shows both inside and out. Here are three main reason to eat for health.

Energy

Ever been too exhausted after school or work to fix a healthy dinner for yourself so you grab fast food instead? Hungry and reaching for that brownie instead of going over to the fridge to get carrots because you just are too tired to think about it? Skipped working out again because you needed more sleep? Without energy, it can be truly difficult to make the right choices regarding your diet, let along maintain an exercise program.

When you choose processed, high fat, high sugar foods over fresh, natural foods, you are going to come up short on energy at the end of the day due to your blood sugar level fluctuating and also due to the lack of vitamins, minerals, and other nutrients to keep your body going. Eating healthy makes it easier to have the energy to have willpower.

Cognitive Function

Along with more energy, eating a balanced diet will also help you think more clearly throughout the day. Just as a car engine needs a steady supply of quality fuel to keep running, so does your brain as it processes the demands of everyday life. Protein like chicken and complex carbohydrates like brown rice keep the fuel in your brain (glucose) running on an even keel, so you don't experience a sudden moment of forgetfulness, fuzziness, or spiciness that can be a result from poor eating habits.

Appearance

Dry hair? Brittle nails? Splotchy skin? All of these are the result of nutritional deficiencies that occur when poor food choices are made consistently over time. Sugary foods not only do not supply any nutritional value, they can even block other nutrients like Vitamin C from being absorbed. Processed foods like white bread tend to cause the blood sugar level to elevate, causing inflammation throughout the body, including the skin. A lack of essential fatty acids, like those found in salmon and walnuts, shows up in dull hair that breaks easily and nails that split or crack.

When losing weight, it's important to remember the goal is not just in the numbers. It's in the way you feel, how you look and how you think, too.

The Importance of Protein in Weight Loss

When you start learning about weight loss, you see the word "protein" come up a lot. And while we are familiar with the term, not many people actually know what it is and understand the important role it plays in weight loss.

What Does Protein Do For Your Body?

The word comes from the Greek word protos, which means first, and points to the critical role it plays. Proteins are groups of chemicals which do many things: they allow the body to send signals so you can see, hear, think and move. They help your body make other chemical compounds that help digest food, create new cells, and build muscle. Protein also helps keep you fuller longer, which in turn is perfect when you are trying to cut back on calories but don't want to be bothered by hunger pangs.

Where Do We Get Our Protein From?

Since it is an essential nutrient which means your body doesn't make it, you must get it from food. Protein that is found in other animals is similar to our own protein; our body recognizes it more readily and incorporates it more easily. Nutritionists call this type of protein 'high quality protein'. Meat, fish, poultry, eggs, and dairy products fall under this category, but eggs are considered the most useful protein to the human body.

You can also get protein from plants sources like grains, fruits, vegetables, nuts, and seeds, but those sources have smaller amounts and are not as easily assimilated. Because these sources are incomplete, you need to eat foods from other categories like grains and meats to make sure you get the complete set of proteins your body is looking for.

Why It Matters For Weight Loss?

Recent studies in weight loss point to the important role of protein. When we diet, we lose weight but often times we are losing exactly what we don't need to lose: muscle mass and bone mass. We just want to lose the fat! Scientists have discovered that eating higher amounts of protein and lower carbohydrates results in diminished appetite and higher metabolism, meaning your body is burning more calories just doing its normal thing. And the weight you are losing is fat, not muscle.

How much protein and what kind of protein should you include? Protein should make up about 30% of your daily calorie intake. Your primary sources should be cottage cheese and eggs. You can also eat red meat, pork, fish and chicken. Be sure to incorporate some at every meal and snack to help with suppressing the appetite and maintaining muscle mass.

What Are Processed Foods?

The term 'processed food' is spoken a lot lately, but what does it really mean? Simply put, processed foods are any food that has been altered from its original, raw state.

Now, with that being said, there are several different levels of processing. It can be as little as peeling the skin from a banana. Or it can be as extensive as white flour bread where wheat has been stripped of its natural outer layers and then ground into a substance that has additives, fillers, and other artificial chemicals combined with it to create something that definitely didn't get plucked fresh from the ground.

What's So Bad About Processed Food?

The more processing you have done to your food, the less healthy it is for you. While processed or manufactured foods are hygienically safer and have a longer shelf life, they also are missing key nutrients that keep your body healthy.

For example, fresh pineapple has an amazing amount of vitamin C. So does canned pineapple. But the fresh pineapple has active enzymes that, along with the vitamin C, provide a healthy array of benefits you can't get from canned pineapple. The vitamins are absorbed more readily because there are in a more natural state. In canned pineapple, the fruit has been altered due to the high processing temperatures in canning cause nutrients to pass through the digestive system instead of being assimilated. And quite frankly, the taste of canned pineapple, while good, could never hold a candle to fresh pineapple. That sweet, fresh taste is your body telling you there's good stuff in what you're eating.

That being said, we live in a world where fresh food is not always possible. And, if we're honest with ourselves, sometime the processed foods taste way better, even if they are not good for us. So what are we supposed to do in those circumstances?

You want to consistently strive for getting half of what you are eating at every meal to be as close to its natural state as possible. That means whole grains and raw or slightly cooked fruits and vegetables.

If it's difficult to reach that level, the next step is to try and get that portion of your meal from frozen foods. Foods in this state still have nutrients because they have usually been flash frozen, a process which minimizes the loss of vitamins and minerals.

Last on the list of is refined grains and canned fruit and vegetables. While still a decent source of fiber and few vitamins, they have been processed to the point of being mostly unrecognizable by the body.

What Is Fiber and How Can It Help With Weight Loss?

You hear a lot about fiber in connection with losing weight. While it is not a magic cure-all for dieters, it is a pretty big weapon in the battle of the bulge. So what is it and how does it help you lose weight?

Understanding Fiber

Fiber is that part of a plant that our bodies cannot digest and passes through our bodies without contributing calories. Fiber comes naturally in two forms: soluble and insoluble. Soluble dissolves in water and insoluble does not. Both types of fiber are found in fruits, vegetables, nuts, whole grains, and legumes.

The difference between the two is how they react in the body. Soluble fiber, the type that dissolves, forms a sort of gel in digestive tract as is passes through, taking it with it some cholesterol and also slowing down the absorption of sugar - a healthy activity for your blood sugar levels as the less rapid pace keeps it on an even keel. Soluble fiber can be found in chia seeds, oat bran, peas and beans.

Insoluble fiber is the type that won't dissolve in water - it just kind of hangs around. But it does have the ability to absorb water, so it ends up holding it, much like a sponge. As it travels through your intestines, it acts a lot like a sponge, too. It mops up certain types of carcinogens that cause cancer and is very helpful in getting bowel movements working again. Insoluble fiber can be found in wheat, corn, oat bran, nuts, and the skins and peels of many fruits and vegetables such as apples.

How Fiber Aids Weight Loss

So now that we know what it is and what it does, let's get to the big question: how does fiber help you lose weight? Four words: it fills you up. For a long while. Studies show when volunteers eat 300 calorie meals with 10 grams of fiber, they stay fuller longer than if they ate 300 calorie meals with no grams of fiber. The sense of satiety comes from fiber expanding in the stomach as well as the effect it has on digestion: it slows it down, causing your stomach to empty out slower than normal, in turn making you feel hungry further on down the road than what you would normally expect. This is a big win for dieters. Eat less yet still stay fuller longer? What's not to like about that?

What Is Nutrient Density?

Which food choice do you think is better for you – French fries or a baked potato? They are both vegetables. They both have been cooked. But the baked potato has less fat and calories and if you eat the skin of the potato, you are taking in more vitamins and minerals. So it would be safe to say the baked potato is more nutrient dense.

Nutrient density refers to the level of vitamins and minerals present in the food. And when you are dieting, you want to make every bite of food count as far as nutrient density. The more nutrients you take in, the healthier you are and the less you crave the not-so-healthy foods. Fortunately, the majority of nutrient dense foods are low in calories. Let's take a look at some of those foods and how to incorporate them into your diet.

No matter what kind of diet you are on – Atkins, South Beach, Paleo, Weight Watchers – they are all going to emphasize nutrient dense foods that are high in water content and low in calories. In other words, lots of vegetables and fruits! These two food groups have the most in terms of how many vitamins and minerals they pack into their structures versus other foods. Apples, carrots, spinach, and kale are all examples of low calorie foods that pack a nutritional wallop with little calorie counts.

So why not potato chips? It's made from potatoes, right? That's a vegetable. But in this circumstance, the potato's water content has been replaced with fat content and along with it, a good portion of nutrients. You end up with something that began as a healthy potato, but got processed into an altered food that barely resembles what it started out as. It's now higher in fat, calories, possibly sodium and definitely missing a good chunk of its minerals and vitamins. Definitely not a good food choice when you are trying to lose weight.

Meat, nuts, and seeds also pack a lot of nutrients in their structures as well, but you have to be a little more care when incorporating them into your diet. These particular foods have a tendency to be fat dense as well as nutrient dense, so it is very easy to eat too much. A handful of nuts per day is sufficient to take advantage of the nutrient density without tipping into weight gain territory. The same goes for meat: a maximum of six to nine ounces of day of lean meats mean you are getting the vitamins your body craves without adding to your waistline.

Why Eating Breakfast Can Help You Lose Weight

When dieting, many people are tempted to skip breakfast as a way to cut back on the calories. Scientific studies have shown that avoiding this meal completely backfires on most dieters. Why? There are several reasons, but first and foremost is that you are setting your body's hunger level for the rest of the day. It's hard to keep on a diet when you are constantly thinking about food, right? Well, you can assure yourself of an easier time of it if you start your day out with a high protein breakfast. The reason is simple: when you keep your blood sugar level steady, your hunger level remains steady, too.

The second reason is that, as implied with the term 'break' and 'fast', it's important to break the fast from your sleep state and wake up your body by eating. When you eat a quality breakfast, you literally fire up your metabolism and the rest of your body's functions. This increases your burn rate on calories throughout the day - something that we dieters are working towards anyway.

There are other health benefits, too. When you eat breakfast consistently, you have an easier time processing fat through the liver. Your cognitive levels are stronger throughout the day. Your body will process insulin more efficiently, leading to healthier blood sugar levels.

Now before you start digging out the cereals and waffles, you need to make sure you are eating the right things for breakfast. Think protein and complex carbohydrates, like Canadian bacon and whole grains and fruits. The reason for this is if you eat processed items like white bread, pancakes, cold cereals or waffles, your blood sugar level will jump, causing your hunger level to return with a vengeance a few hours later. You want to focus on food that requires more of your body to digest. Think low fat or nonfat plain yogurt with berries; whole grain breads like pumpernickel or stone-ground whole wheat bread; steel-cut or old fashioned whole oats instead of instant oatmeal.

Don't forget the lowly egg for breakfast! Nowadays, eggs are lower in cholesterol than those of years past; scientific studies are indicating an egg a day has no harmful effects on your own cholesterol when combined with a healthy diet. In addition, evidence has shown those dieters who eat eggs for breakfast tend to feel fuller longer and consequently eat less throughout the day. Bonus for us dieters

Why Experts Say Diet Sodas Are Not A Beneficial Part Of A Weight Loss Program

Cutting calories is an expected part of your weight loss journey, and when you look at the possible ways to reduce caloric intake, choosing diet soda seems like a correct choice, right?

Or is it?

For years, numerous scientific studies have demonstrated the health hazards of regular sugary sodas: tooth decay, diabetes, and of course, weight gain. But believe it or not, new scientific studies on the effects of diet soda are bringing to light the exact same health hazards - including weight gain!

While scientists are not sure as to exactly why the body reacts to diet sodas as if they were sugar-filled, they do have a few theories. First, there's nothing nutritionally redeeming or natural in diet soda. It's a combination of laboratory chemicals combined with water and carbonation. And if the body doesn't recognize what's being ingested or doesn't have the ability to totally break it down to excrete it, it will store it away in fat cells. The more you ingest a substance that it can't break down, the more you will gain weight as your body tries to find storage for the chemicals it doesn't know what to do with.

Other scientific findings point to the disruptions between the taste buds and the brain when it comes to diet soda. When diet sodas are ingested, they seem to signal overeating. It works this way: your tongue receive intense messages of sweetness when you drink diet soda. It tells your brain that it has a pretty big incoming load of calories. So your brain prepares the rest of your body to process the anticipated caloric intake, including releasing insulin, which makes your cells ready to take in energy from the digested food Only with diet soda, you don't deliver on those calories, leaving your body with an elevated insulin level (bad for your body) and your brain thinking there something missing somewhere. So it will urge you to overeat later in the day to make up for that jacked-up level of insulin you ordered earlier.

In addition, those same scientific studies point to diet sodas as contributing to overeating in an additional way: a dulling of the taste buds that detect sweetness, leading to you to hunt down sweeter and sweeter things to eat and drink as you try and satisfy your sweet tooth.

No matter how you look at it, diets sodas don't have a place in your weight loss journey.

Why You Need Antioxidants and A Guide To Natural Sources

The weight loss world has its own lingo and one of the phrases you'll hear over and over again is 'antioxidants'. So, what are antioxidants and why are they so important?

The Science Behind Antioxidants

Antioxidants are plant chemicals, vitamins and other nutrients that help clean up something called a free radical. In chemistry lingo, a free radical means a molecule in your body is missing an electron. This is not a balanced state, so the molecule searches out other molecules to grab that missing electron and when it does, it creates another free radical - another molecule missing an electron. So what does this mean? When you have molecules stealing electrons from other molecules, it leads to conditions like clogged arteries, accelerated aging, and damaged tissues - in other words, oxidation of your body's systems.

Why do free radicals occur? Actually, free radicals happen inside of you with natural body functions, like when your immune system fights off a cold virus. That process of killing the virus creates free radicals. Normally, a healthy body has no problem cleaning up the free radical mess and taking care that other mole cues are balanced. However, when you consistently eat a poor diet, don't get enough sleep or exercise, experience continual stress or come into contact with contaminants like pesticides and other toxic chemicals, the free radicals overwhelm your body's ability to contain them and that's when the damage starts occurring.

Enter antioxidants. These little powerhouses have the ability to scavenge for and destroy free radicals, breaking the chain reaction of instability and reducing inflammation and damage to your body.

Where To Get Antioxidants (Naturally)

While you can supply certain antioxidants with vitamin supplements, they only can do so much. Antioxidants work in conjunction with other bioactive elements like amino acids to do their job, so obtaining as many antioxidants from fresh, natural food is your best bet to controlling the free radical race inside of you.

What kinds of foods have antioxidants? The best ones come from fruits and vegetables - and the more colorful, the better for you it is. Antioxidants can be found in the pigment (the color) of those foods. Strawberries, oranges, lemons, broccoli, blueberries, eggplant, and blackberries are just some of the foods that are great sources of antioxidants. Aim to eat five servings of fresh fruits and vegetables each day to give your body and your weight goal a fighting chance!

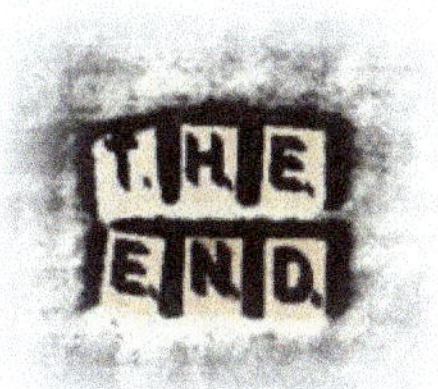